I0441715

Momma's
Chuckles

A Heartfelt and Humorous Journey Through Alzheimer's

Cheryl L. Emery

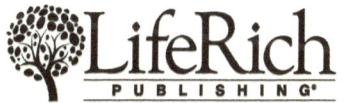

LifeRich Publishing is a registered trademark of
The Reader's Digest Association, Inc.

LifeRich Publishing books may be ordered through booksellers or by contacting:

LifeRich Publishing
1663 Liberty Drive
Bloomington, IN 47403
www.liferichpublishing.com
1 (888) 238-8637

Because of the dynamic nature of the Internet, any web addresses or
links contained in this book may have changed since publication and
may no longer be valid. The views expressed in this work are solely those
of the author and do not necessarily reflect the views of the publisher,
and the publisher hereby disclaims any responsibility for them.

Any people depicted in stock imagery provided by Getty Images are
models, and such images are being used for illustrative purposes only.
Certain stock imagery © Getty Images.

ISBN: 978-1-4897-1607-1 (sc)
ISBN: 978-1-4897-1606-4 (e)

Library of Congress Control Number: 2018902808

Print information available on the last page.

LifeRich Publishing rev. date: 03/23/2018

Dedication

To Momma

I Love You More

Talk to me...let me talk...and then try to redirect my mind.

If I'm angry - it's not really with you ...

It's my anger with myself, the situation that I can't understand ...with the disease that is stealing my life away. Please don't take it personally. Always Remember How Much I Loved...Love You. It's harder for me than it is for you.

~ C. Emery

Prelude

The journey through Alzheimer's, with a loved one, is a difficult one. More and more of us are deciding to not let them go on that journey alone.

Their pain is your pain. Their sadness is your sadness. Their anger is your anger. Their confusion is your confusion. When they no longer have their memories, we share ours with them. Sometimes there is a glimmer...a sparkle, that reaches out of their darkness. There's a happy, shared memory...a smile...and a "Momma Chuckle" that makes it a little easier.

As my beautiful Momma went further and further away, I made it a point to write down happy, silly, amusing things she said. It helped, that day, to tame the disease that was taking my Momma from me. I also knew, that when my Momma left this Earth, I would need to remember those wonderful moments when the disease did not take my Momma's witty humor and insight from her. I would need those Momma's Chuckles for the rest of my life. Momma and I would both beat Alzheimer's because of the wonderful person she was. My Momma really was – A BEAUTIFUL, GENTLE, LOVING SOUL.

I miss her every day, but Momma's Chuckles help to bring her heart back to me, when I need her the most.

I hope that if you, or someone you know, is on this most difficult journey, take the time to cherish and note those special moments. It has been the best coping skill, for me, to weaken the Beast of ALZ.

My sister, Karen, summed it up, "You don't let go of the memories... you just start to let go of some of the pain." I, often, wondered, if I was actually strong enough to do what my Momma so rightly deserved. It was a blessed honor to care for her. Even given some of the repercussions, I would do it again, in a heartbeat.

Momma beat Alzheimer's on July 9, 2016. She never knew that she lost her husband of 54 years on 4/14/12, her daughter on 8/31/14, her grand-daughter on 3/5/16 or many of her sisters and brothers (or her parents who passed away long ago.) Momma, now, has ALL her MEMORIES back. Thank you, God.

I started "Momma Chuckles", on Facebook, before I lost Momma... for moments like this.... when the pain feels unbearable. I REMEMBER "My Momma", when she was herself, not the disease. That is what will be my MEMORY of Mary Haudenshild Jacobs Kirkwood. I love you, Momma. This book is for you.

Karen: Karen Kirkwood; youngest daughter of Momma

Mike: Mike Emery; son-in-law of Momma; Cheryl's Husband

Sam/Samantha: Samantha Simms; Caregiver and Friend of Momma and Family

Stashia: Stashia Alvarez; Caregiver and Friend of Momma and Family

Earl/Pop: Earl Kirkwood; Momma's Second Husband; DOD 04/12/12

Ted: Ted Jacobs; Momma's First Husband; DOD 10/21/56

Sandy: Sandy Junker; Momma's middle Daughter; DOD 08/31/14

Jaimee: Jaimee Kirkwood Reese; Momma's Granddaughter; DOD 03/05/16

Traders: Traders Seafood Steak and Ale, Chesapeake Beach, Maryland

Stephanie: Stephanie Holland; Caregiver and Friend of Momma and Family

Doug: Doug Junker; Momma's Grandson; Sandy's Son

Keno: Momma's 4-Legged Companion; Cheryl's Chocolate Lab

John: John R. Grube; Momma's "Third Good Man"; DOD 12/05/05

Poston's Fitness For Life: Dunkirk, Maryland

*Denotes a corresponding picture in the picture section of this book.

Now for some of Momma's Chuckles...

We were at Traders restaurant... Momma looks around and says, LOUDLY, "Wow! I'm the only WHITE one here!" Then she points at her white lemonade - the rest of us had diet coke or tea.

Momma thinks it's 4:15 a.m. and has gone to bed...angry that I tried to explain that it's 4:15 in afternoon...says I am trying to keep her up all night...hasn't been to bed...Guess the honeymoon's over :(

Momma has made her bed every day, forever. All is smoothed out and hanging just right. The pillows are in their place...fluffed and ready for that night. This morning, I noticed the blankets... the pillows...are somewhat crooked and flat...the bedspread is not straight and slightly laying on the floor.... it's ok, Momma.... I made it look like it "always" has. Love you, my beautiful Momma.

My sister, Karen, said, "I have my class on Hickory Lane, Huntington, Md....I said, " I don't know where that is...wonder where it is?". Momma says, "Huntingtown." :) I love my Momma

While sitting in the doctor's office, a woman walks in with a long dress on...Mom says, LOUDLY, "she can wear that as a dress or a tablecloth!"

While on the way to Traders, my husband told Mom that he just got back from church. I asked him how it was. He said it was about God and Jesus... Mom said, "I wonder if anyone knew them there." :)

My husband was messing with Mom, saying "women are dumb"... When she asked him again what he said...? He changed it to "women are smart"... Mom says, "It's good that that's finally come out!"

My day started with Momma letting Jehovah Witnesses in..... :)

*My dog has bitten heads, tails, feet, butts, etc. off most of my yard figurines.... BUT Mom says I am wrong and it just requires putting them back together.... Mom says this one is now perfect again. It has tails where legs should be...heads where arms should be...but it's perfect.

Momma...Momma... She was shuffling thru some Mega-Million tickets that were laying on the table...She asked what they were. I told her that we might be millionaires and we could go anywhere we wanted. I asked her where she'd like to go.......She said, "To bed." Love my Momma

Mom's ROTFL thought.... Without being too graphic... offensive... Momma thinks certain men's part should have a bell that rings when things arise....wahahahaha...I was driving, and I almost ran off the road!!!! Then she says, "There....there's your laugh for the day"!!!! Love my beautiful Momma! (Yes, Sandy.... I know... I know... couldn't help it.)

*Momma just says, "Hey...I'm missing someone" ... (looks around). I asked her who.... She says, "Earl... where is he?" I told her, "don't know...he didn't tell me, but he should be back shortly. "Pop", her husband of 54 years, died 4/14/12. (Several months earlier, Momma realized, for a moment, he was gone, while talking to my sister, Karen. She asked, "What did we "do" with him?" Karen, gently and with a heavy, heavy heart, explained to Momma.) Even loved ones deaths, they can't remember. One of the very few "blessings" of ALZ.

Three of my grandkids were here, and there were at least 6 "other strangers", too, "stealing all Momma's stuff".... throwing all of it in a "train car" (dumpster)...throwing away "her perfectly good things that she could fix" - though wasn't sure what "that" ...or "this" ...was - But you DON'T throw good things away...EVER (the oldest girl of 16 kids that always had someone that needed it... or at least could fix it...) (None of it was Momma's).

As we had a busy day, Momma should have had a horrendous day/night. A little bit of agitation was just fine with me... and again attests to Momma's strength and love... just below her own personal hell. I love my beautiful Momma. You just never know what to expect.

Conversation in the car... I was making. "Smartass" remarks.... My grandson says something like "well that's pretty 'usual' for you Gramma" (smiling). I laughed and said I also have a Smartass grandson. :) He then said it must be hereditary. Momma quickly says, "well, I'm not a Smartass!" I started laughing and told them that would make her a dumbass!!! Momma just laughed and agreed.

I said, "OH MY GOD...." Momma says......"He's mine, too!!!"

Momma wants to know if there really is "HOLY" shit????

Momma is wearing her new clothes that we got yesterday...I was afraid she would insist they didn't belong to her today. Only problem was that I was looking for my glasses....finally found them ... Mom was wearing them!

I wanted to share how deep a love my Mom has for her "child". As most of you know, Alzheimer's patients, always want to go "home"... As Momma did last night...she took one look at me after I told her I would take her "soon".... She said, "I can see you are sad and tired... It's ok if we go in the morning." I so love my Mom! Those moments are so precious.

Out with the "childproof" and in with the "Momma-proof"! :)

My sister, Karen, and I were sitting on the front porch... with the frog that strangely appeared every night for months. :) Suddenly, the porch light went off....Pitch black outside. I quickly said..."the light must have burned out"...Karen opened the door to check whether the switch was up or down...it was down (i.e. "off")... I said, "You know, it's a sign"...., "Sign of what?", "....a sign someone is visiting us" (from Heaven)....both of us became apprehensive and "spooked". About that time, Momma came out disoriented....she had been asleep. Karen said, "It still was a sign.......a sign to let us know Momma was up!" :) Geez! It really was a little spooky. Karen didn't see anyone when she first opened the door.... :) We THINK Momma turned it off...probably.

While driving Momma to a doctor's appt., she kept saying, "Wow! Look at all that traffic! Geez...I don't know if I could drive, anymore, around here!" I had to smile...Momma was looking at a car dealership parking lot! Love my Momma.

Mom and I had a good trip yesterday from Florida. The coming "home" wasn't as smooth. She loved the new bedroom (special thanks to all that did an awesome act of love for Mom and me... you know who you are). I thought we were smooth sailing but... The waters turned rough...and then stormy...then the gale winds and waves almost overcame Mom and me. After a while the storm calmed...mostly because no matter what...at least for moments in time, my Mom's deeply engrained love for her child, took over. So, now, we are going to be living in "MOMMA'S HOUSE", using "MOMMA'S FURNITURE".... Whatever it takes to make Momma feel "at home.... In 'HER' home." :) Even "that man" (my husband) can live with Mom and me.

Mom woke up last night and we held each other til we fell back to sleep.

She is now up...drinking her coffee, eating her yogurt...has taken her meds...though as she often does, asks what they're for and me giving my usual answer... "For what ails ya, Momma! "

Momma just said she doesn't remember having "THIS house" for long... doesn't remember having this many trees around "HER house"... Wants to know who has lived here...told her "you and I have always lived here...with some other family members..."

Momma wants to know if she also had a husband or someone... I said, "Yes, Momma." Then says, she's lost half her mind. I told her, "me, too, Momma. Me too. But if you have half your mind and I have half my mind, then together we have a whole mind...and we'll be ok."

I've been "eyeing" a gorgeous, two-seater, black convertible, 2009 Sky...showed Mom and told her that it ought to be "our car". She said, "But there would be no room for our boyfriends!"

Momma stopped, abruptly, at the kitchen door. Mike was following right behind her. He said, "Momma you are gonna need to keep going." Momma says, "Well, next time, you need to honk!" Love my Momma.

I just can't get past the "it can't be true" thoughts. (My beautiful sister, Sandy, took her own life, while Momma was in her care in Florida. I then brought Momma to my house in Maryland.) It takes my breath away over and over. It just CAN'T BE TRUE! I NEED MY SISTER!!!! I try not to cry in front of my Mom - she may be the "lucky one" right now - she only worries about how sad I "look"... wants to know what SHE can do to help ME!

When I get home, do not ask me why I have pieces of Kleenex all over my clothes from the wash.... I'll get this all figured out. Momma forgets, and so do I, that she always puts Kleenex in every pocket.

Sandy....Do NOT let me forget to give Mom her nighttime meds again...she wasn't a happy camper...and YOU, more than anyone, knows what happens.

*Sandy was right...I shouldn't have gotten Momma this damn Christmas Cactus...Mom has moved it so many times that it should be receiving FREQUENT FLYER MILES!!! (Sandy mentioned this to me a couple of months ago...).Guess one of the "things" about Alzheimer's, is the need to constantly "relocate" your stuff that you don't want to forget to take "home". Momma also had what we called her "hobo pack". It could contain just about anything...and not always her stuff. She would "pack it up" to go "home"...over and over...and over. She usually used her housecoat...and tied the sleeves together to hold everything in.

Again, Momma was asking where Pop was....I told her he's probably at work....she said she didn't think so...I said that maybe he's working at the church...she said probably not....then I said, "maybe he's at the gym..." She says, "As long as its Gym...and not Jane!" Love my Momma. I miss my Pop.

Momma was having a tough morning this morning. I needed to take my niece, Jaimee, and her daughters back to Va. I decided to take Momma with me. We drove to Virginia and back today...6 hours of driving. Momma did pretty well until the last hour and a half home. Her anxiety and talking was on overload so I was holding her hand....talking...redirecting...therapeutic fibbing my ass off... She looked at me...then my hand...then the windy roads and said, "You need to put your hand back on the wheel...you're making me nervous!" :) Love my Momma

"Momma you are so pretty!" Momma says, "Yep been this way for years!"

While driving to Traders this evening, Mike says to watch out for deer – "they sleep during the day and run at night..." Momma says, "They're men, aren't they?"

When we would see a dead deer on the side of the road and she would say "oh dear!" (My sister, Karen, and I now do this. Guess it's one way we keep Momma with us.)

When Momma and Samantha were to go off to play Penny Bingo at the Sr Citizens' Center... :) She wasn't very happy about it, but I didn't waiver. When she came to me and said, "Why are you making me go out of here?", with tears starting. :(I told her I wasn't making her, and she'd have fun...meet some new friends.......she said, after looking at Sam, "I already have a friend."

Momma wants to go "home"... I told her it was just too nasty and slippery out today...She starts singing, "Please help me I'm faaaalllling..." by Hank.

Momma asks, "What is this CRAPISON?"...Samantha Simms and I burst out laughing....Momma was drinking CAPRI SUN!............ guess she got the "R" in the wrong place. :) Love my Momma

I was helping Momma get her bathing suit on ...told her everything had to come off. She took everything off....looked at me and said, "you're not gonna make me go on the stage now, are you?"

Stashia (Another awesome caregiver and friend to all), asked Momma if she knew Stashia grandma's name. Mom says, "Yes... Grandma!"

Stephanie (A substitute caregiver and friend) was sitting, dancing to Momma's Elvis' Jailhouse Rock...Momma looks at her and said, "Oh I got more than that!"

*Momma had 16 brothers and sisters....she was the oldest girl. She's always been able to name all, in age order. Trying to redirect this a.m., I ...asked her to name them....trying to help, I started her with "Bob....then Mary....who's next Momma? Mary....then?" Momma says, "MARY...and JOSEPH."

I was talking to Momma in bed, saying maybe we ought to get up and walk. She says yes... if her clothes don't fall off. Told her that's OK, I'll put her robe on her...Unless that'll fall off too. She says, "if it does, I'll just "pass the hat"!!!!!

Sam came outside as Momma and I were sitting on the porch... Sam says, "Hey!". Momma says, "Save your hey (hay)....you might marry a horse someday!"

We were driving thru Rosehaven (a small town in Maryland). I was trying to redirect Momma when I saw some beautiful yellow roses. I pointed then out to Momma and asked her what she thought they would do if I picked one (me thinking...COPS, etc.) Momma says, "They'd probably ask if we wanted another one".

We were blowing bubbles on the front porch (Sadly, Momma, initially, tried drinking and blowing without the bubble wand...). Then when the bubbles kept landing on her...she says, "Look! They LOVE me!!!"

Taking a shower... Apparently phone rings...Momma answered it... but they had already hung up...it takes Momma awhile to figure out which button to press.... She brings me the phone in the shower.... She says someone named "**CID**" is calling. (CID=Caller ID).... Told her to leave phone with me and I'll answer when they call back...few seconds go by... she brings me her IPAD....so I can answer, when they call back... told her it only plays her Elvis music...few seconds go by... she brings me the TV remote....AND, YES, you can let the dog out!

On Traders deck... Music is loud.... Momma was ahhhing and oohhhhing...and looking uncomfortable....Then I realized what she thought they were singing.... I explained the song was "Play that FUNKY Music...." and "Uptown FUNK"!

"Where was I before here?" "Florida, Momma." What was I doing there?" "Visiting Sandy, Momma." "Is she still there?" "Yes, Momma...she still lives in Florida...she still lives in Florida." :(

We put out the hummingbird feeders... told Momma they fly up from Sandy's house in Florida... Momma says, "or any place else they can get a ride from."

Out of respect, Mom's caregivers would call her Miss or Ms. Mary. One day, she looked at Stashia or Sam and said, "That's MRS MARY!"

In Walmart. I wanted to try an outfit on. I said, "you can come in with me." (meaning Momma into the fitting room). Momma turns to this man standing there and says, "I think she means me...not you!!!" Man was cracking up...I was dying.

As I'm totally undressed from the waist up, after trying on an outfit in the fitting room.... Momma looks at me and says, "you gonna go back out there looking like that?"

I reached for Momma's hand (her's are always warm) and told her my hands were cold....her's were too, she told me. She said her face was, too....I told her my nose was cold...her's, too. She said, "Guess we ought to put them in somebody else's business!"

Momma having some sharp pain on her left side around her ribcage. I was feeling the area and asking Sam what organ, etc. might be there...I asked, "What could possibly be there?" Mom says, "Your hand."

In trying to redirect an agitated Momma, I asked her what she thought of DC legalizing pot. She says, "It's just like cigarettes." I told her that wasn't really true. She says, "Oh yeah...there's that flying high part."

My Mom is hilarious...she was watching a game show... The question was "What helps you sleep better at night?"....Her answer was, "Going to bed!"

I asked Mom if she knew whose birthday today is...she asked, "What day is it?" I told her October 5th. She said, "Sandy's...." Then she asked me. "Where's she living now?" "Florida, Mom...and it's Doug's birthday today, too." "Oh yeah, Doug's birthday, too. How old is Sandy today?" "Well, Momma, she's 59 today..." Momma says, "Well...and I thought I was old!"

We were listening to the song "Christmas Island" by The Andrew Sisters. I said, "Yeh, Mom...you've been to an island...I'd spend Christmas on an island...gladly! ...and you've been to Hawaii." Momma says, "Yes, Havii" :) I said, "You've been to Cancun, Switzerland, Germany, England...." Momma says, "Yes...and France!" I asked her any other places?" Momma says, "OHIO!"

Told Mom...geez lost my Bluetooth again... Momma says, pointing to her missing tooth, "yeah... me, too! I don't know where mine went either!"

We were talking about Thanksgiving and "passed down" family recipes. I asked what was "in" our family recipe for Sweet Potato Casserole......Momma says, "Sweet Potatoes"...

Keno (my dog) was looking out the window...Momma says, "You expecting company?"

Mom kept saying her ice tea tasted like water (we finally figured out it was unsweet tea...not her usual sweet tea.... So, we kept adding sugar...after about 4 tries we gave up.) A minute went by and Mike asked how her water was....she said, "It tastes like ice tea." Love my Momma

National anthem comes on the car radio at noon... Momma says,"Sorry... I can't stand up"...but then sings every word...every time....until she couldn't any longer. (So now, I sing it for her, whenever I'm in the car, at noon.)

Driving past Birdsville, MD., Momma sees all the horses... "This should be named Horseville...I don't see any birds!"

Trying to calm down Momma while waiting for doctor. Tried hugs, music, candy, videos and more meds...nothing was working. Finally, I asked her if I could sit on her lap. Momma says, "No....you'd probably piss on me!". Love my Momma. (This may have been the first time, EVER, that she uttered a "bad word." Unfortunately, this was mild for future words.)

Stephanie was trying to get Momma to eat the last of her oatmeal. "Ms. Mary...Ms. Mary...look at me..." Momma looks at her and says "aaaahhhhhhhh, yikes!!" And then bursts out laughing! Love my Momma

Momma Chuckles: (if easily offended... skip this one:). Playing the name game outside.... using alphabet for girls' names starting with.... A is for Ann...B is for Betty...C is for Cathy....etc...up to V is for Vickie....Momma's turn for W........"What's a girl's name that starts with "W"? Momma says, "Whore"....... love my Momma

Hurray...Momma didn't mind her new "Fitbit" bracelet that the Sheriff's Office put on her. "Project Lifesaver" ...so if Momma goes walking "home", we can bring her back. Radio frequency specific to each individual. Why aren't more families using this service from Office of Aging? It can also be used for children at risk. Gives a little peace of mind during the cold winter nights...actually anytime.

Momma wants to go home. I told her she can't go home but has to come to my house to get better. She said, " What... So, I can clean your house?" Love my Momma

*Pizza came...Momma says it's looking at her! (Two pepperoni eyes!) Lol! Love my Momma

Momma says. "I'll need to go to the dentist...what do I need to take? I said, "Just your teeth!" Momma says, "but I'll need to take an arm and a leg, too..........because that's what they'll charge me!" Love my Momma.

Sam said to Momma, "Did you sleep good last night?"...Momma says, "yes...until I woke up." Love my Momma

Momma Chuckle: (sorry...only family may get this one...) All the time, Momma and I go thru the "ditty" of me saying "Momma Mia" ...ME a Momma ... YOU a Momma, too. YOU a Gram-momma.... ME a Gram-momma too...YOU a Great Gram-momma...ME NOT a great gram-momma........well Mom "one upped me" this morning with...."and ME a MEMAW!" (my kids' nickname, they gave her when they were very little…a long, long time ago!) Love my Momma.

*Momma was in the hospital and noticed her "DNR Bracelet". She asked me what it meant. Since she wanted to go home, badly, I told her it meant "Do Not Return".

I just told Momma she's a nut.... she says, "Yes... I live with a lot of them!" Love my Momma

Bought another 50 of Elvis songs for the IPAD that Momma's been singing to all afternoon....Samantha Simms gave Momma her 5 p.m. meds.... Momma says, "What's this...something to shut me up?" Love my Momma

Dag... Momma just introduced me as her FRIEND, "Cheryl Emery" :'(

I told Mom I was driving around topless today (I have a convertible). She says, "Were they clapping?" (my "girls")

After a rough last couple of hours of OCD behavior.... I decided it was time to get Momma ready for bed. Sometimes it's a challenge to get everything off...when I told her, "Let's let the girls go free", she says, "Ok .... but they better be here when I get back!!! I'm gonna need them later!" :)

Was watching my beautiful Momma this morning from the front porch on the video monitor...she looks so frail, confused and lost... she's trying to remember how to get out of a bed...there's a guardrail to prevent her from falling out again... she crawls out "my side"... Still with a little pain from her fall in Florida...she picks up the pillow from the floor...starts "making the bed" like she does every morning...and has done probably most every morning since she was a child. She stands in front, unknowingly, of the video camera.... and..... Rips a giant fart.... a toot. (Passes gas - for those of you that don't fart!) I crack up laughing...laugh each time I remember...YEP... I know you did that, Sandy...we both know our Momma doesn't do things like that...but sometimes is BY a dog or grandchild that does :) It was hard, feeling like I was invading her privacy, but I needed to be able to go out of her room and not worry that she had fallen or was needing me.

Thanks, God, for all your help...and letting me keep Momma awhile longer. Be patient my beautiful sister, Sandy... It's still my turn.

Mom (in hospital): "When are YOU leaving?" Me: "I'm leaving when you leave, Momma." Momma: "Well... Let's GO!!!"

Stashia told me that she was helping Momma get dressed. Keno (my dog) was in the room, so Karen said, "Momma, Keno just saw your butt!" Momma says, "Well, he didn't whistle!" Love my Momma

*Momma is much better this morning, after visiting the ER for a foot infection. But...she just wants to know why someone drew on her foot! (It looks like Sandy's Florida, so I'm sure she's telling me it was good I took Momma to the ER.)

Couple days ago, my husband Mike, Momma and I were leaving from Traders. Mike hit the accelerator to get out into oncoming traffic. Momma says, "WOW! You almost threw me out the door!" I said, "Yep! Me, too, Momma!" Mike said, "Well if I did, I would've left you laying there!" Momma says, "Well....SOMEONE ELSE would've come by and picked us up!" Love my Momma

To the nurse at the doctor's, I explained that Momma isn't patiently waiting... well Momma is but ....ALZ is Not.

*Momma keeps "taking a walk"... she's looking for her home... surely, it's right over there.... She walked up and down the driveway up to 30 times a day.... looking for her house. We don't know how she did it. I'm glad I let my neighbors know about Momma. They had to bring her back...when I was too long in the bathroom.

Momma says her food is cold.... asked Traders server to put in microwave for 30 secs (and I'm not sure if it's cold or not... feels warm to me....). A couple minutes go by and Momma asks me how come I have a plate of food and she doesn't.

"Groundhog Day" movie.......lived by Momma and me :(

Just gave Momma a hug....and then gave her one from Sandy. Momma says, "Where is she?" I told her, "Where there's sunshine... and it's warm." :'(

Ok...whatever works...Momma's been struggling...can't get her out for a redirect..........put "On Demand" ....she's calmed down and watching the crazy movie "Airplane".... wahahahah....who'd a thought? :) It reached a point, where Momma was a "part" of whatever program she watched. :(

While Momma was in Florida, I'd talk to her sometimes a couple of times a day. Being her oldest child, I think she usually knew me and could usually be calmed by me. Finally, headed there to give my sister a break, I'd drive to the airport early in the morning and be in Florida by 10a.m. BUT...Momma always thought I just lived down the road.

Momma Chuckle: Karen was changing a really, really, bad, poopy diaper of her grand-daughter's. (We are dying from the smell.) Momma says, "I think that's some of the stuff from MY purse." "yep....maybe Momma, I said"... Everything "belongs" to Momma!

Mike was outside. He came inside and put his hands on Momma's face.... she said, "Phew....be glad you didn't have to pee!"

In hospital emergency room ... She wants to leave now. I told her she must be patient... She says, "that's what I am being... laying in this bed... A patient!!!"

Dr. was checking Momma's vitals, etcetera. He said, "out loud" to medical scribe, "No slurring".... Momma says, "of course not... I haven't been drinking!" :)

Mom just said she has never seen a pink turkey before. I told her it was a ham. She said "Okay".

Momma watched me close the front door to encourage Eddie (a neighbor's dog) to go "home"...about that time the clock started striking the hour with chimes...Momma says, "Look...he's ringing the doorbell!"

"Momma Chuckle" (she's full of 'em this morning!) - Mom says, "I guess My Mom and Dad got something special on Christmas Day... ME!!!" (Her Dad delivered her at home on Christmas Day... thus the name Mary.)

One of my daughters sneezed...Momma says, "You sneezed so hard I think I saw something fall off the Christmas Tree!" :)

We were just sitting on the front porch, enjoying the weather. Momma says, "I think I need to relax so my boobs will get smaller."

Samantha and I were talking about someone that had recently died.... She asked me what he died from...before I could answer, Mom says, "His heart stopped." :)

Sam looked outside and said, "Ms. Mary...looks like a delivery for you!" Momma says, "A baby!??" (She had gotten flowers.)

Geez...Momma got an escort out of Trader's at lunch...luckily, the sheriff didn't believe she was being held against her wishes...or that she was being kidnapped by Sam. The other patrons were uncomfortable when she kept saying, "Help, me...help me!" :(The sheriff took her to Sam's car. Momma got in without a word. Clarification: Momma <u>asked</u> for the escort :) We are eating dinner at Traders tonight, as usual. :(

At Traders... Standing in omelet line. Momma was in front of pastries... Lady reaching for sweet pastry saying "looking for something sweet" ... Momma says, "well here I am!"

Beware...this chuckle could be offensive.... Momma heard some quite nasty swearing (nope...not from me!). Momma says, "Do you suppose there are "Father Fu**ers?"

Samantha asked Momma how she slept last night and how many sheep she counted... Momma says, "I don't know...I just went to sleep...and they laid down and went to sleep, too. They said, 'Baaaaaaa'...which meant Good Night." :)

After going with Sam to the dentist and then to the Sr. Citizens' Center's Penny Bingo, when Momma came in, I asked her if she was tired of running the streets all day...She said, "We didn't run the streets...we rode in the car."

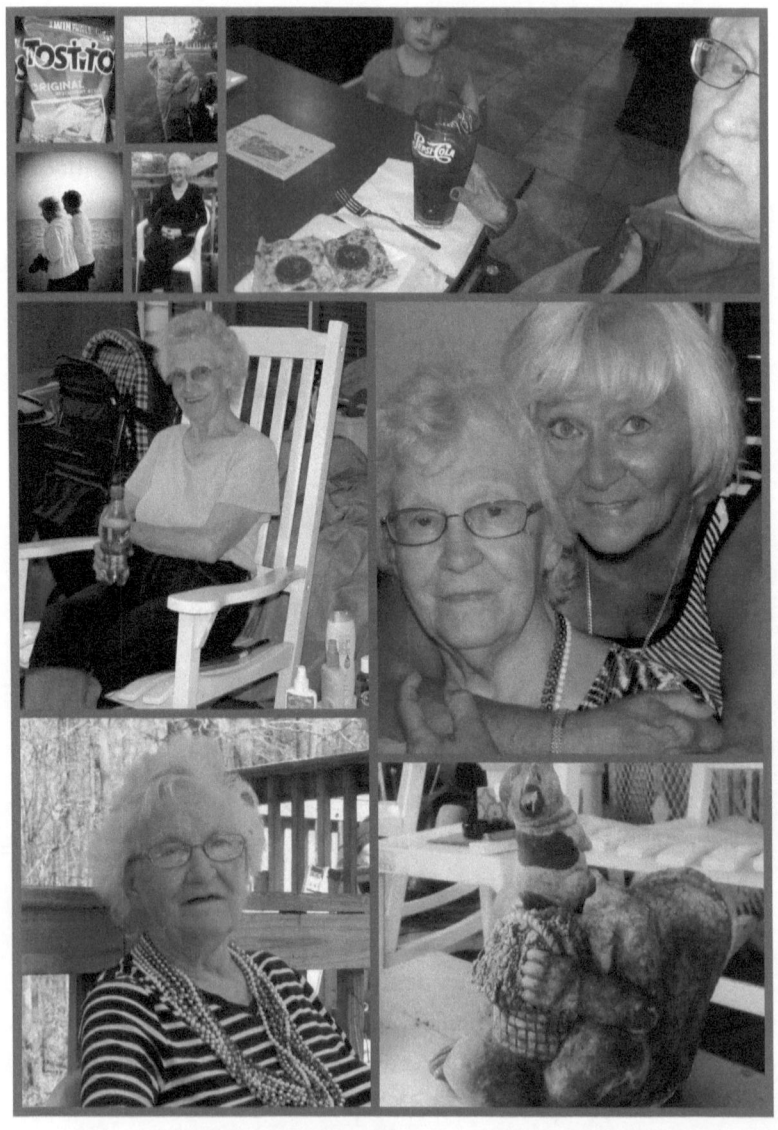

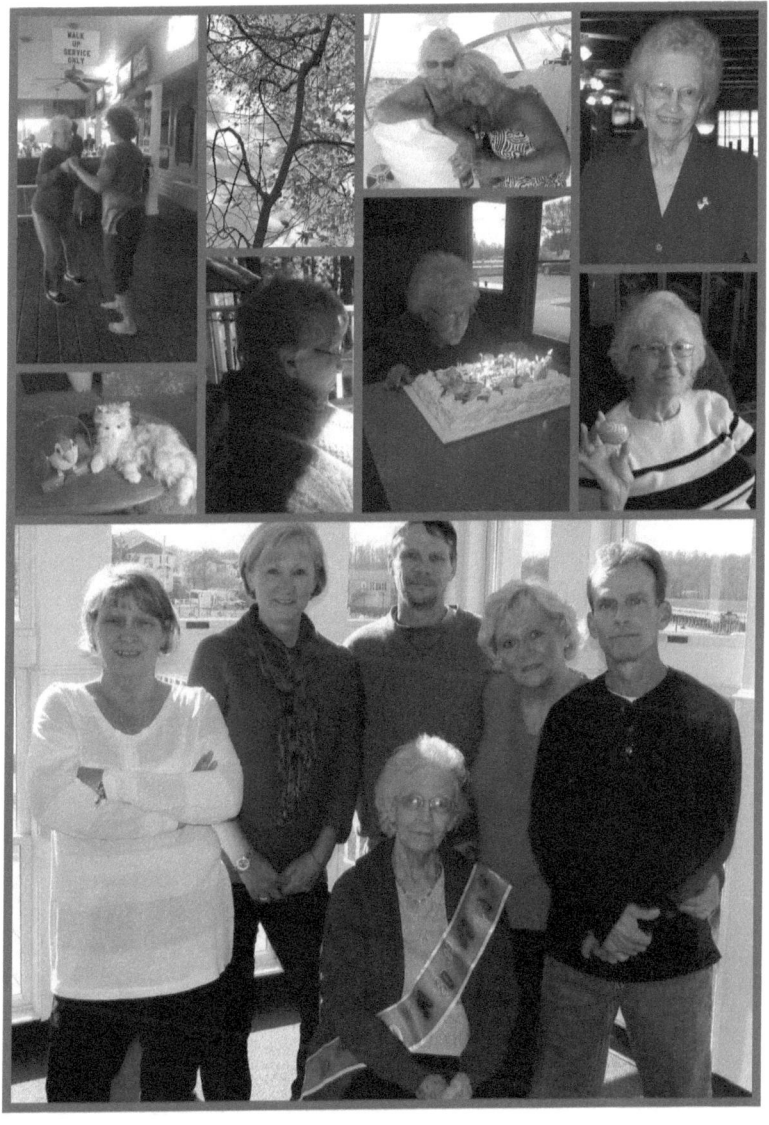

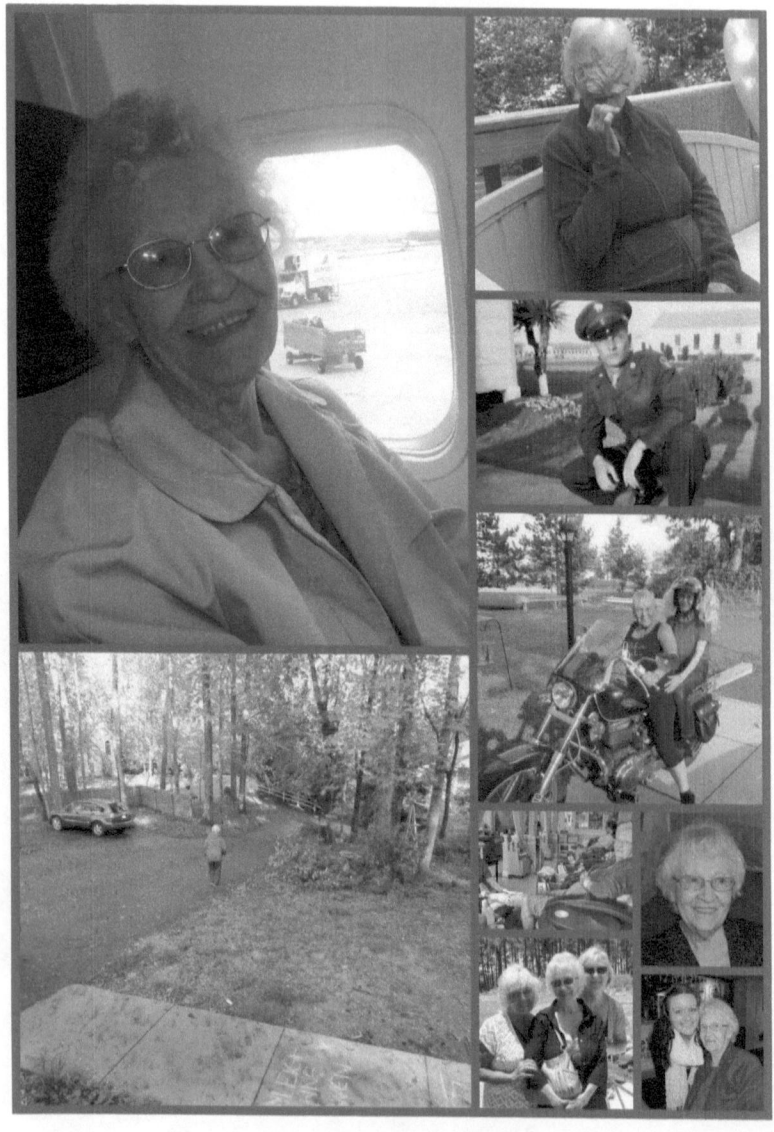

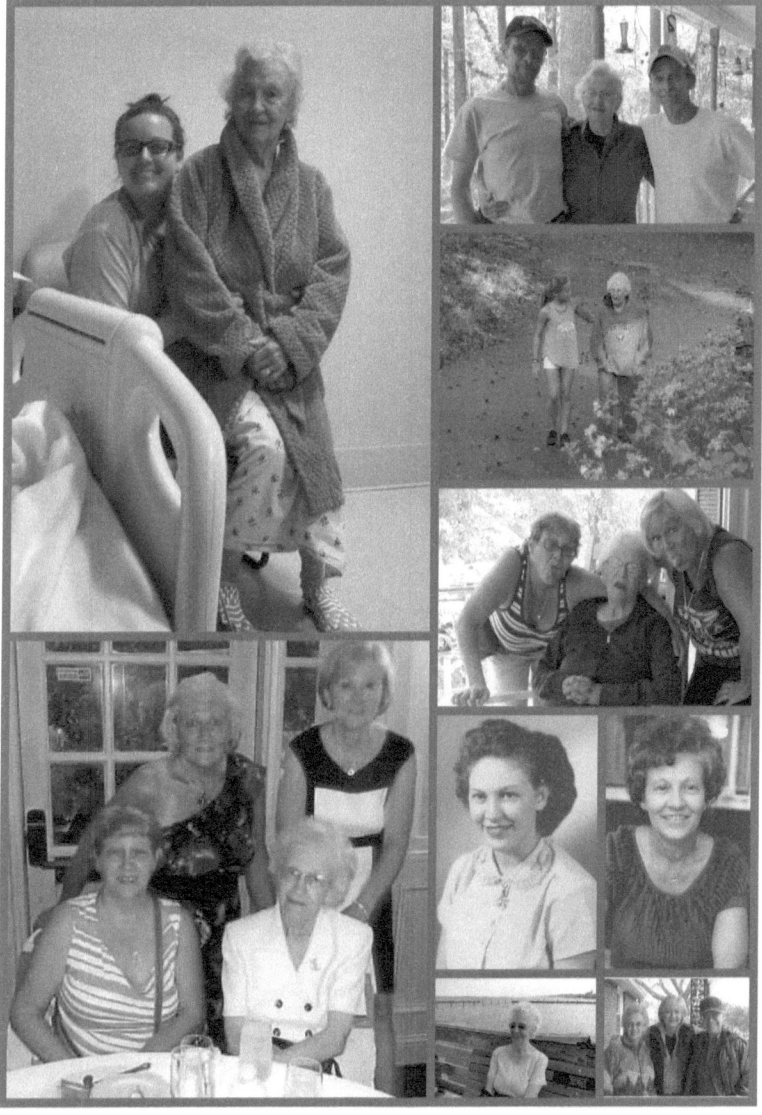

23

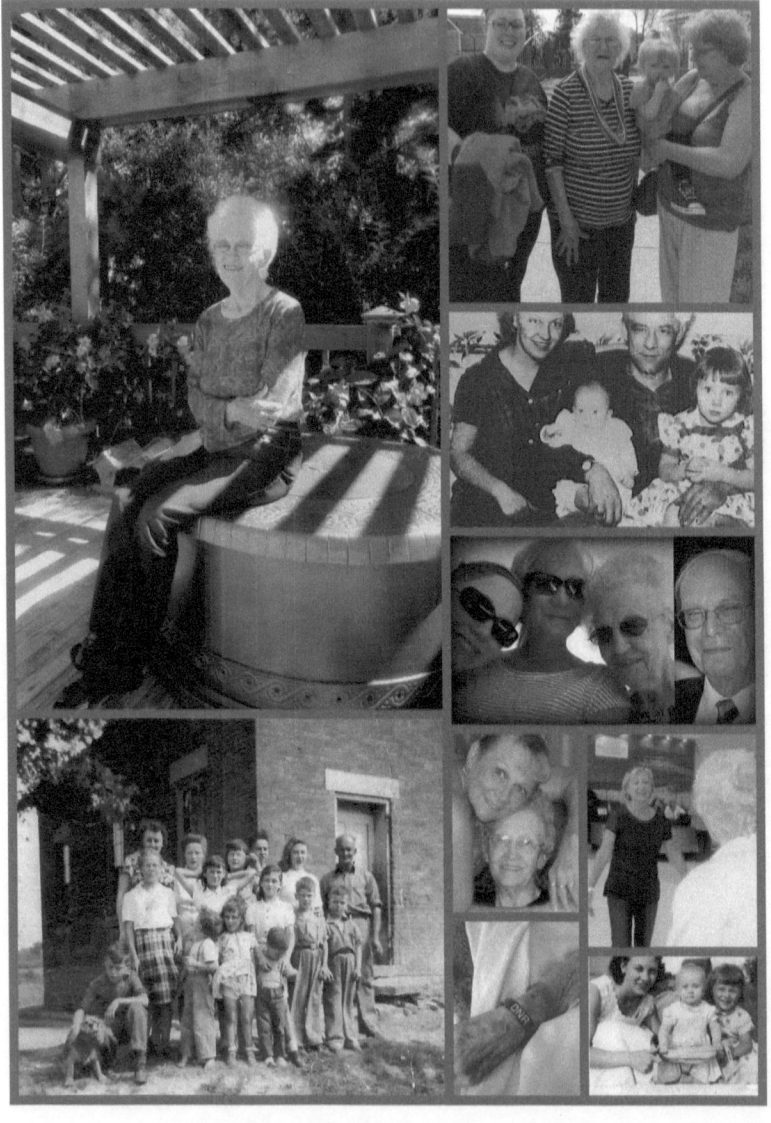

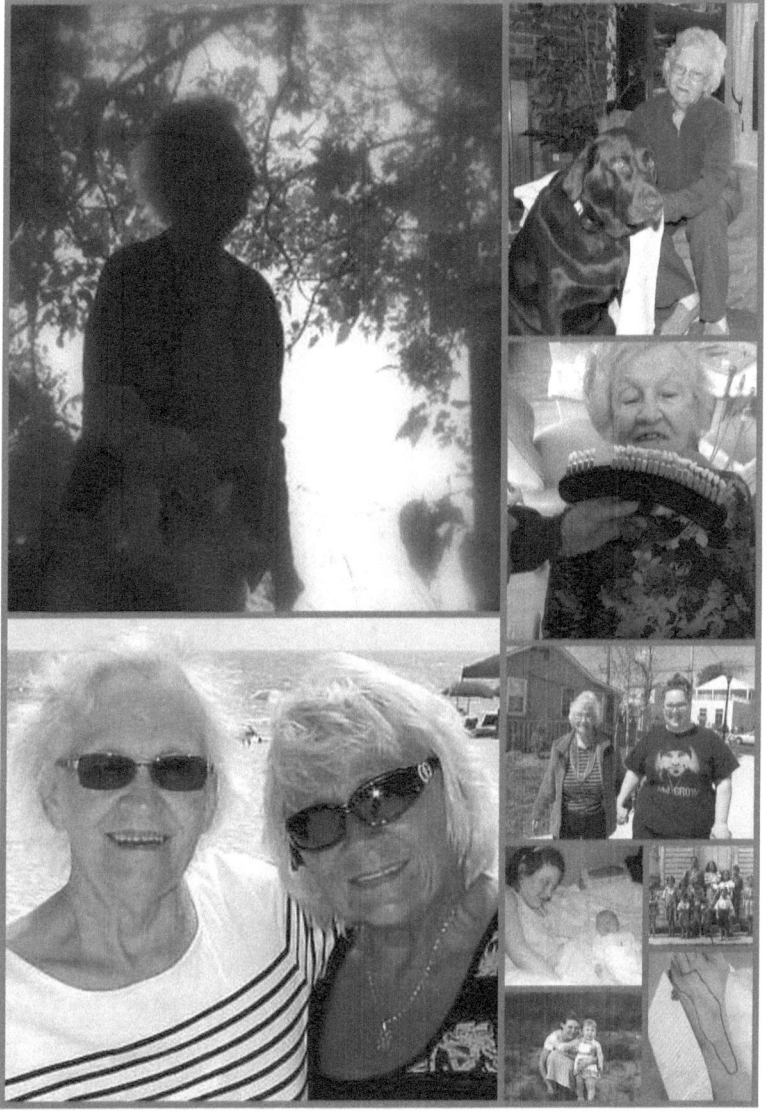

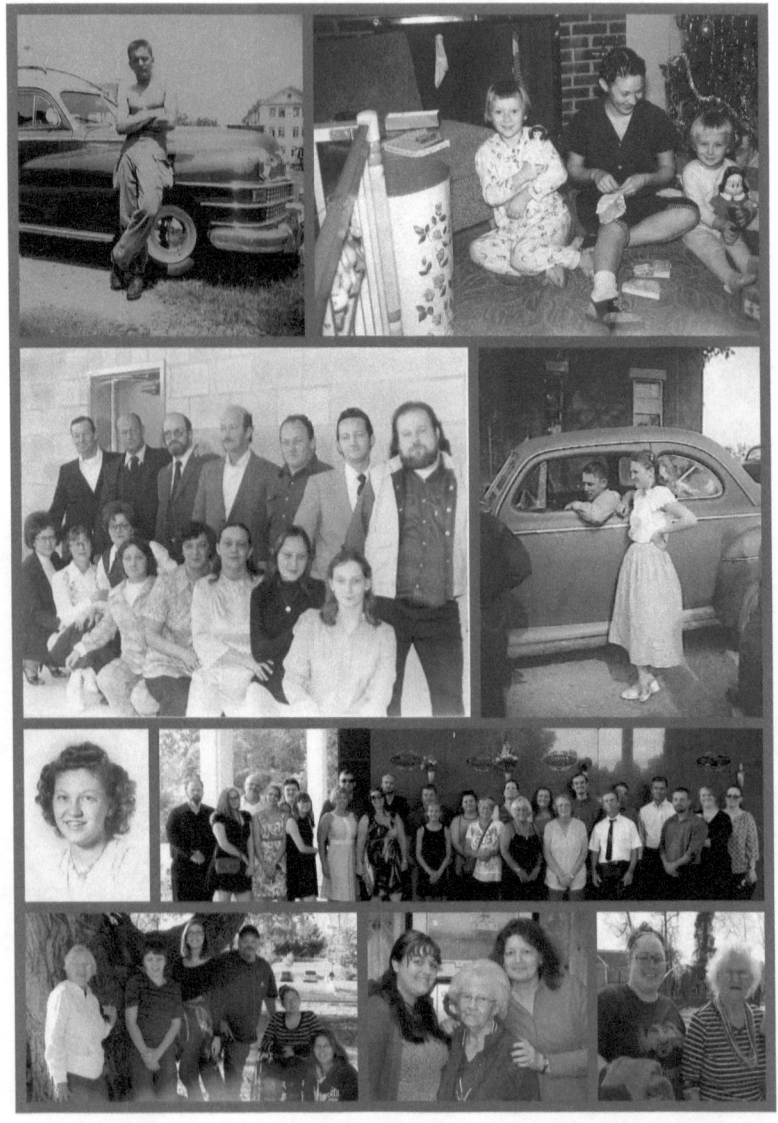

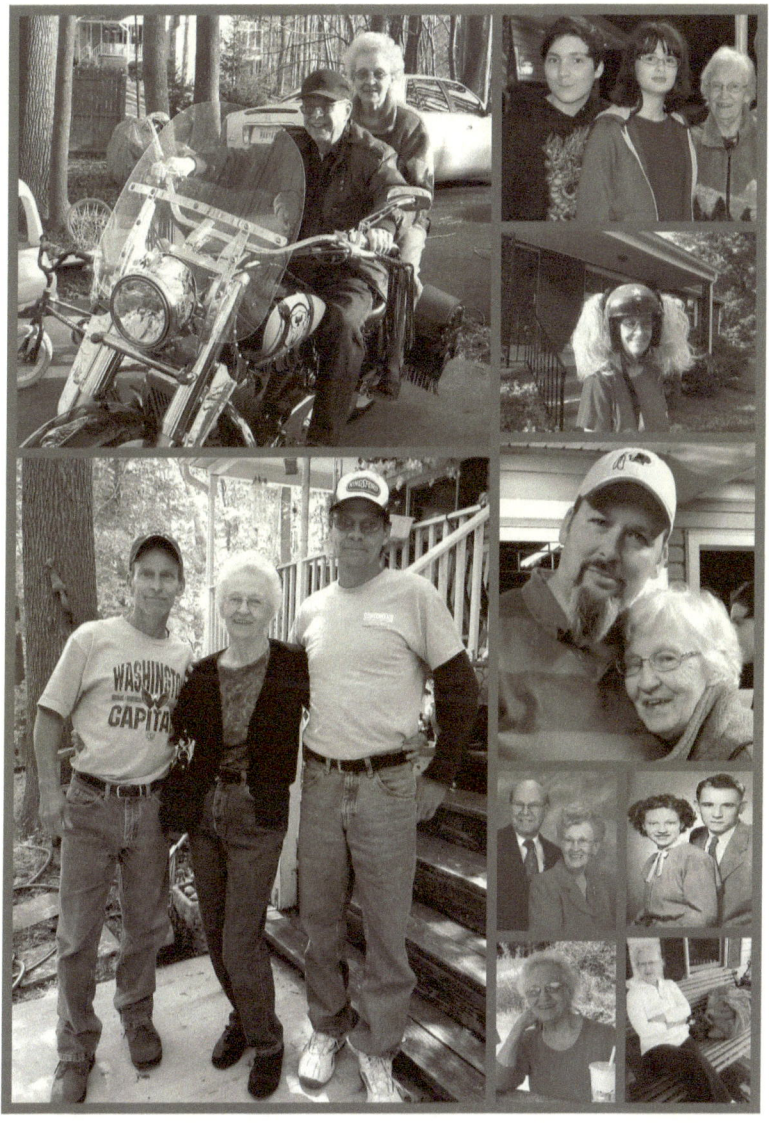

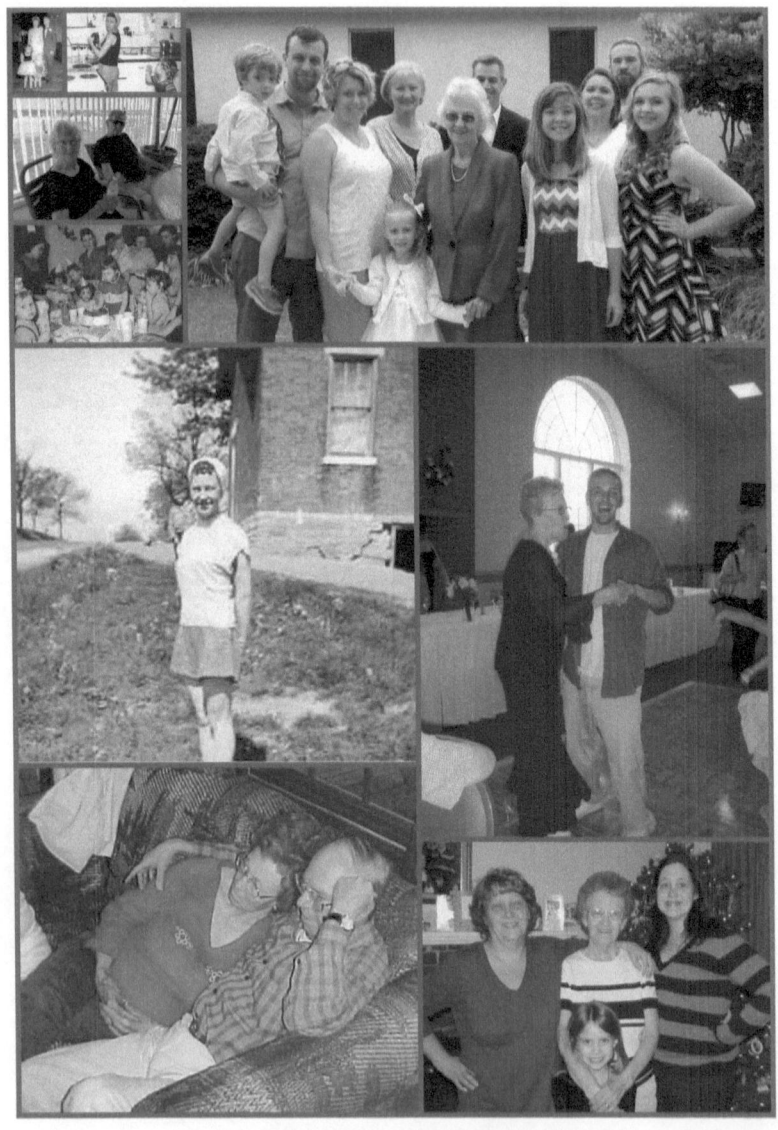

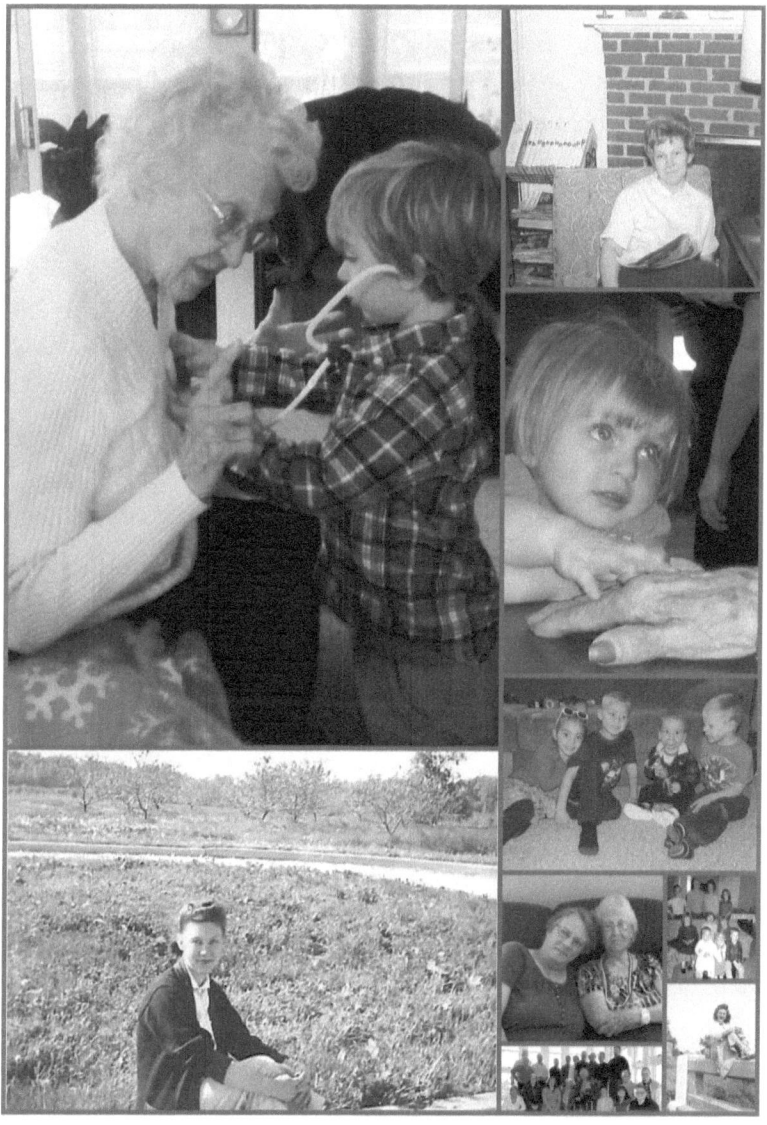

We were talking about family (kids) being around (for Thanksgiving) ... says she likes having them around...asked her how it is when they go home...Momma says, "Wonderful!"

Samantha was just telling me that while she and Momma were driving in the car today...Momma laid her head back...Sam told her "Now, don't go to sleep on me..." Momma says, "I can't...you are way over there." :)

Momma was making "fish noises" (thought she was "talking" to the fish... in my aquarium). Samantha asked her if she was talking to the fish...Momma says "No." Sam asked her who she was talking to then...Momma says, "Myself."...Sam asked her what she was telling herself... Momma says, "To shut up."

Momma wants to go home...told her I needed to go to the gym first.... She says, "What's his name again? Jim? Are you gonna work out...or work in?" (Says she gets "this" from her kids) :) Sorry, Sandy... I heard you sigh that I posted this - shouldn't have left me...I need your supervision :)

I had inadvertently put white socks on Momma...white but "different" ...they didn't "match" - one had "writing" on the toes - the other didn't. I told her we needed to change her socks to match... incase the "Sock Inspector" came... Momma said, "Then maybe he'll bring us some new, matching socks." ...and she didn't really need to match, as she next said.... she was gonna put on her shoes.

I was vacuuming and kept bending over to pick up Keno's dog hair.... I finally turned around, looked at Keno and said, "What's with all your hair all over, Keno?" Mom answered, "Yes...it's HIS... and HE wants to know what YOU are doing with it!"

We were talking about some family members this morning...I said, "they have to be high school or older"...Momma says. "Yeah that's me"...I said, "oh, you're in high school? "..."No I'm the older"...I said what am I gonna do with you? She said, "anything you want, Hun... anything you want."

We asked Momma what she wants for her birthday.... she said, "Another year."

Momma just asked me if Ted is dead. "Yes, Momma, he died awhile back".... (1956 - Her first husband)

Asked Momma if she needed some more coffee...she said, yes. I laughed and inadvertently "lightly sprayed spit on her".... she said, "What are you doing.......trying to make me grow?" Now we are both laughing...I said to her, "Momma, we are a pair of nuts!"..........
.... (you know where this is going........) and Momma says, "You know that's not possible, don't you? We are both girls!" :) Love you, Momma. Thanks, Sandy for leaving her with me

Momma is drinking her coffee out of a cup that says, "United Way 2001 Campaign Together We Raised $100,000" (yes, I have old cups...but this one is big and requires less refills.) I reminded her to eat her bowl of oatmeal sitting next to her and not let it get cold.... She asks, "Ok...so if I eat this oatmeal will I get "$100,000?"

Helping Momma get dressed...she "thinks her girls are getting bigger"

After driving Mom "home" for the past 45 minutes ...we drove past Lake Erie in "OHIO" (Chesapeake Bay) and past Myrtle Ave in "OHIO" (We live in MARYLAND.). Mom decided since we were having a hard time finding our house (in OHIO), we'd stop at that place over there - Traders....... Says we can try again in the morning because she doesn't want me driving after dark.

Momma was watching "Price Is Right" and the woman was repeatedly jumping up and down......Momma says she needs to stop doing that because, "It will sour her milk!"

We are eating at Traders....sister Karen leaned over to Momma... laying her head on her shoulder. Momma lays her head on top of Karen's....Karen says, "I'm tired." Momma says.............. "I'm Mary."
Love my Momma

Momma asked, "How old am I?" I told her, "You are 81 but you'll be 82 on Christmas Day." "No wonder I'm tired!", Momma says :)

Yesterday's "Momma Chuckle"...we were going into Traders Seafood Steak and Ale yesterday (as we do almost every day), and Momma read the sign, "Traders"...she said, "So what are you gonna trade me in for?" I told her I wouldn't trade her for anything in the world.

Momma did not get the "time change" memo.... but it'll get dark "sooner" and we'll work on the "no, Momma, it's NOT bedtime yet...yes, I know it's dark outside..." :)

Ok...got Momma some winter boots and gloves...but couldn't find an "appropriate 81 yr. old's hat"...I couldn't deal with the tassels on top... also picked up some gates for the hallway and the "up" the stairs... doing well and feeling accomplished...... until Momma puked :(

Told Momma I needed to go pick a few things up today...but can't remember what they were...but, hopefully, that they'll come to me before I go. Momma says, "Good...then you won't have to go get them!" :) (if they're gonna "come to me").

Told Momma, I hoped the gas I was having this morning was gone before I went to "Poston's Fitness For Life" studio. Needed to get a new workout routine......she said, "can't you put something up there that plays music?"

Ha-ha...Momma "got me today"...we ate at Ledo's for lunch, after getting Momma's "NEW Drivers' License"........well, exchanging old for new ID Card. (Though she hadn't drove for years, she insisted that she STILL had a license and could drive if she wanted!) We got into the car to leave and Momma said, "Oh, no... I forgot my purse inside!"...."Glad you remembered before we left!" She started laughing when I saw her purse sitting on the FLOOR of car......then said, "Haha...Gotcha!" :)

Momma just told Keno he couldn't have any of her coffee because "you'll run around in the yard like you had a BEER!" Love my Momma

WhaHaaHa! Helping Momma get dressed after her bath...told her to put the "ladies in".... She says, "Ok, girls.... settle down and get in there..." (This may be a post that Sandy is not "happy with"... told her to not leave me unsupervised)

Momma just asked, "Where did Sandy go?".........told her she's still at work. :(

Momma just said, "That's the best bath I ever had!" (Actually, it's the ONLY bath she "remembers.")

Trying to make my phone stand up so we can listen to Sandy's music.... Mom says," it can't stand up....it doesn't have any legs."

Momma just said the sun's gonna come out now.... SHE just turned it on :)

*Momma shopping... guess what she called Tostitos....LOUDLY :)

Mike had a dumpster, to clean out basement junk, delivered. Momma says "well, don't throw anything of mine away!" I told her I'd make sure that doesn't happen but "I may just throw myself in it!!!" Momma says, "Well YOU belong to ME!!!" So, I laughed and told her she was right... and I'll stay out of the dumpster :) Love my beautiful Momma.

Mike just said to a server at Traders, jokingly, to stay away from that end of the table because they are all gay...Momma says, "We are???" :)

Sandy once told me of an episode when she and Momma were shopping. A salesman came over to help them. As he was walking away, Momma says, LOUDLY, "I think that guy was a queer! (No offense but Momma was from a different time.)

HeHeHe...just had an "evil thought" :) Wonder what would happen the next time a telemarketer called...I handed Momma the phone :) I know YOU have wondered the same thing!

Yep... I think we'll go to the County Fair for a while. If we are lucky enough to see any of you there...please remember...Momma doesn't know her beautiful daughter, Sandy, is now an angel.

Ha...looking for my glasses after my shower.... Finally found them. :) Apparently, Mom and my eye prescription is as close as we are.

Momma just pointed a banana at me...told me to get my hands up!!! Love my beautiful Momma

Ooppss...? moment of some clarity??? Mom just asked where Earl is (Pop died 4/14/12) and, as usual, I said I thought he went to work... about 5 minutes goes by and she looks at me and said, "Earl doesn't work. He didn't come here with me..." Finally, I told her I musta been thinking of earlier this week...my mind gets confused...." :(

Dag, Momma...I was looking for my stuff......I gotta remember to check her purse. :) Found things I didn't even know were missing yet. I love my Momma.

WhooHoo...shower was a success (don't ask me if my legs are shaved...)! WARNING FOR THE FUTURE: If you see me running butt naked down 5th St., please throw me a towel...Mom may have gone for a "walk" again.

Sitting on front porch in rockers...I told Mom to "sit right here" so I can get her some coffee... So, she got up out of HER chair and sat in MINE :)

I helped my beautiful Mom get dressed before I left (again, thanks God for having me do this because Mom needed help out of her confusion and with only 2 males there, this could've been a problem. :) Anyway, I made the mistake of bringing Mom the wrong bra to wear. We laughed, and I said, "yep...God gave 'us' the big boobs...." She laughed again and said, "Well, don't tell Sandy!!!!"

* Momma says she didn't write "SHIT" on an Easter Egg but that Samantha did :) Momma said her handwriting is better :) Love my Momma

We are all laughing so hard at Momma....with Momma. Momma says, "They're back there saying, look at those crazy ladies.... They're NUTS! OH, NO... We don't have any of those!". Love my Momma

After an hour and half waiting to see Dr., Momma is "starting" .... :(says, "I didn't come here to spend the night!"

While sitting on front porch, Stashia threw Keno his newspaper chew toy...Momma says, "he must want to read it!". Stashia says, "Maybe.". Momma says, "He may need glasses!". Love my Momma. (Keno was amazingly perceptive to Momma's and our needs...more so than many humans.)

*We're at dentist redoing the impression for Momma's new teeth. They get out the "matching guide" and Momma says, "Well... that's not gonna fit in my mouth!!!?" Love my Momma

Momma says, "Stop making me laugh.... I'll blow bubbles out my nose!"

At the doctor's office... After the umpteenth time...Momma says, "Did you sign me in?". We said "yep"...Momma says, "Cheryl should go up there -motions sticking chest out- and tell them we're waiting." Asked her what they would say to that...she says, "Have you been here before?". Love my Momma....hope this is the new meds...

We were asking Momma what each of our names were. Momma says, "Cheryl Louise, Karen Denise....and what's your name?" (Looking at Stashia). Stashia replies, "Stashia Marie." Momma says, "initials are SM.....that means Smart Woman." (It just dawned on me that she transposed the M to a W.) Love my Momma

A woman was in a hurry...Momma says LOUDLY, "She must have to go to the bathroom!". Love my Momma

Mike is driving us to Momma's doctor appt... his IV machine started beeping... He said it says, "high pressure".... Momma says, "Gas!!!" Love my Momma.

We were sitting in the dr.'s office...Momma asks if they are gonna call her name. We said yes...she said, "does that mean I need to lick my lips (and look sexy)?"

Momma just said, "I'm losing it..." Told her I wish I could do something and sorry she has to go thru this. She said, "don't be sorry...You haven't done anything wrong...." Love my Momma ....
Hate HATE HATE ALZ!!!!

Keno was outside...and started barking...Mom said someone is outside...Mike went to check...it was the mailman delivering a package.... Keno is barking...barking... in the meantime...As Mike is walking out the front door to get Keno and meet mailman, he says, "Come here, Dummy!" (meaning Keno) ...Momma says, "Is he talking to the mailman?"

Momma just picked up a jar of cashews sitting on the table...looked at Mike and said, "Are these YOUR nuts?".......(Mom and I both are cracking up!!! Mike not so much.........wahahahahah)

It's dark outside even though it's not 6:00 yet. Out eating dinner (yes, at Traders) ... Momma says, "You know what I think we are?" No, what Momma? "Night crawlers!"

We pulled in the driveway...Mike got out of the car...but Mom just sat there...not opening her door. I finally said, "Ok, Mom, we're home...let's get out." Momma says, "Oh, this is your house?".... Yes, Momma. She says, "Oh, I thought we were just dropping him off at his house."

After getting Momma's hair done last night, she was sitting on the couch this morning and I said, "Wow, Momma... you look like a movie star...". Momma says........"Which one?" :) I told her she looks like Betty White :)

As always, I tell Momma she already gave me money for her lunch before we left home.... Usually she looks relieved... Today she says, "You're Kidding me..." I assured her it was true.... (She was always worried that I was "treating" her. I would try to make sure she had some money in her wallet...but it always disappeared...)

I was bending over the hearth looking thru some old picture discs... Momma "goosed me"... as I jumped I said, "Hey, why'd you do that?" She said, "I just wanted to see how fast you could go up the chimney!" :)

Dag...just found my cellphone in Momma's purse

I just asked Momma if her coffee was getting cold.... she said, "No.... it's getting gone." :) Her cup was empty.

Karen was getting her granddaughter, ready for bed last night.... I looked at her... and then Momma... and asked, "Should I put her down first?" (We laughed until our bellies hurt.... you could take "PUT HER DOWN" several ways...and we laughed at each one.)

Decided to put Momma in backseat for safety, on the long ride to Fredericksburg, Va. Unfortunately, her legs would not hold her body up....so she slid down to the floor of the backseat....and front seat was up as far as it would go. Her hips were "stuck" between the backseat and front seat. Karen crawled over her grand-daughter to help un-wedge Momma :) Problem was Karen and I were laughing so hard that I was afraid we'd have to call the fire dept. :) Did I mention we both had to go to the bathroom by the time we were done? :) THEN as soon as we got Mom up and in the front seat.......... she had to go to bathroom, too. I love my Momma.

Yep...."36-hour day" is right – Read the book!

Momma says, "Karen, can you tell me what I'm supposed to do with these?" Karen says, "Do with what, Momma?" Momma says, "THESE......my hands and butt". I say that I think she meant to say hands and feet.... Karen insists that no... she meant to say BUTT....because she pointed to it :) and stuck her feet straight out ("and THESE!") Karen's and my stomach's hurt from laughing so hard...and try to make sure Mom doesn't realize we are laughing at what she said....... Love my Momma. (It's ok...she was happy to see us laughing...she doesn't remember what she said...) UPDATE: Momma just asked if...when... she could take her finger out of her nose!!!! Oh, we're getting light-headed from laughing!

Momma only "forgot me" for a few minutes of times. She "wanted" Cheryl...even when I wasn't there...we even laughed, and Karen became "Cheryl #2"...Stashia or Sam became "Cheryl #3".... for that I am thankful. It was my biggest fear...that Momma would forget me. :(But, it was the hardest, when I heard her pleading for Cheryl to help her...and there was little else I could do.

*Momma always wanted me to paint my large country porch RED, WHITE and BLUE!! (Samantha and Stashia will attest to this!). Soooooooo... we painted two wooden benches, in honor of MOMMA, after she passed away! (Wish we had done this sooner, but she sees them now!) All the walking up and down my driveway by Momma (we still don't know how she continued to do), we moved the bench closer and closer so she (and we) could sit down and rest. Towards the end, we used the bench to rest just getting her out of the car. Well, Momma.... Karen and I are going to give you YOUR red, white and blue bench!!! Now, every day, Momma's Bench makes us remember her love and smile. Miss my Momma!

Ok, Momma...we got your message loud and clear. Karen was outside trying to identify songs that Momma would like at her funeral. I was inside doing the same thing. (Momma was a very big Elvis Presley fan.) Karen came in to have me listen to one she liked ("If We Never Meet Again This Side of Heaven"). I was listening to this song ("Take My Hand Precious Lord") and as Karen walked into the room, the song she was listening to CHANGED into the one I was listening to.!!! This song was NOT on the list of songs Karen was looking at...NOWHERE! I think Momma just let us know that she is Ok and made it to Heaven. Apparently, this is a song she wants!!! :) Love my beautiful Momma...still helping us.... I could envision Momma beaming, as she had once again helped in another one of our life's hardest moments. We could picture Momma, Pop, Sandy and Jaimee in heaven looking over us.... Sandy was saying, "Well...it was MY idea." Jaimee then saying, "REALLY? No, it wasn't. No, that's not true. You're making that up Aunt Sandy." ...Sandy then saying. "I did not...... I wouldn't make that up... That wasn't me!..........Well...IT WAS my idea".......then Jaimee saying, "Grampa...that's not true......nobody listens to me" ... and then Pop saying, "Ok, enough girls...knock it off and go to bed!!!!" Momma then says, "Oh, Earl. They got the idea from me." :) Even being "sent" Reverend Faith Lewis, to be here, today with us, was a gift from God. Ask me about it later.

My niece Jaimee's 33rd birthday was Tuesday. I can see them all in heaven celebrating with her. Sandy, of course, singing Happy Birthday, as she always did; and like my daughter-in-law said, "With a Hallmark Birthday Card in hand :) ...or five... Pop having made the beautiful cake, as he did so many times for all of us and Momma smiling and singing along and always happy to be with her family.

"Your loved ones' lives don't end...they change (in Heaven)."

*Acknowledgement: My Momma told us she had "Three good men." This confused us. Momma had only been married twice... Ted and Earl...but she insisted...THREE Good Men. After doing DNA research before she died, I discovered that I was actually "an only child." Her "third good man" was my previously unknown, birth father, John. They had stayed in contact throughout their lives, for 70 years, with letters and cards, etc. I now have, at least, five more "new" half-brothers and two more "new" half-sisters – one deceased, to add to my two half-brothers and two half-sisters – one deceased. I love my Momma.

Her "Notebook" ending was different than the book/movie, but she had a good, happy, full life. She is missed and loved by all.

Special Thanks

Momma's "caregivers" (and friends...to Momma and her family) are greatly missed everyday as well. Samantha Simms, Stashia Alvarez...you have my heart forever and Stephanie Holland for helping whenever needed. They became such a big part of Momma's and our heart wrenching journey. They loved her as if she had always been theirs too. They, without hesitation, took care of my sister, Karen, and I as well. They will always be in my grateful heart. Thank you.

Janie Jonas and Josh Jonas loved and cared for Momma, in Florida, at Sandy's house. You helped my beautiful sister, Sandy, so much. Me, as well, in the darkest part of my life. I will always remember your love and compassion in the deepest part of my heart. Thank you.

Windy Junker, a niece, that grew to love Momma from the day she came into this family, cared for her, with love. She shared her two little ones with Mom in Florida, too... until her ALZ actions became more difficult to explain. Thank you.

Momma's oldest grandson, John Thompson, my awesome son, has always loved her and it showed even more when he cared for Momma. He and other family members were here with Momma on her final day on Earth. For that, I will always be grateful. Thank you.

To the Traders Seafood Steak and Ale (restaurant) Family, I thank you for your love and patience with my Mom. Repeatedly warming and cooling Mom's food, without question, was so appreciated by her caregivers and me. Her repeated cries of, "I want to go home… will you take me home? They are holding me hostage and against my will. I am being kidnapped…" You handled graciously and with your hearts. A true "family restaurant." Thank you.

To Poston's Fitness for Life, I thank you for giving me a way to release my stress and worries. Thank you for helping me be "strong enough" – both physically and mentally. There are days you kept me sane by exercising away the sorrow. Thank you.

So many people connected with Momma and helped her (and us) those last days. I wish I could name them all…but YOU know who you are. Thank you.

ALL of you helped keep Momma here for me, until it was finally her time "to go Home". I don't know what I would've done without each one of you. The old, "It take a village…" comes to my mind.

Momma passed away in my living room…in her own chair, surrounded by loved ones. For that I am grateful to God. Thank you.

To all, I am eternally grateful.

Thank you.
Cheryl

Momma looked beautiful and at peace. Thank you, God!

Love my Momma.... and.....

"Momma............. has left the building"

My beautiful Momma WON on July 9, 2016 ...Alzheimer's LOST!

Mom

You started your life on a Christmas Morn,
It was in the year, 1932, that you were born.
Your Dad held you close, as you came into this life,
Your Mom just smiled - for she was his proud wife.
Many, many children later - that you helped raise,
Even this very day, they shout out your praise.
For each new sibling – sixteen totaled all of you,
Trained you to be a Mom – so nothing was new.
You met a young man – he was handsome and tall,
You were happy for a while until he received heaven's call.
But out of that time - two little girls came to be,
That would be daughter Sandy....and also would be me.
You were lonely and then around you did look,
A shy guy you smiled at - a new chapter in your book.
He was quiet and had little experience in so many things,
But before very long, you were wearing his ring.
The four of us moved from Willard to just outside of DC,
On a dead-ended street, so much growing you did see.
First there was Michael ... Mark... then Karen came to play,
Our family kept growing - your love there every day.
We had others that stayed with us and challenged your heart,
We had a full, large family right from the start.
Cousins, sisters, brother and friends were welcome in our home,
You made sure they were loved and never felt alone.
Piano, dance, horns, clarinets, flutes – lessons for each of us,
You made sure that we were busy – which was always a must.
There was Church, Boys Club, Campfire Girls and Cub Scouts,
Just teaching us what love.... life.... and family was about.
As we grew up and built our own lives around here,
We used all you taught us – lessons learned – so less fear.
You taught us to love, be honest and do our best every day,
None of us would want to live our lives any other way.

Mom, you have always been our gentle soul and guide in our life,
You always supported us in decisions we made – wrong or right,
You were quiet and constant in showing us the way,
But we all knew that our hearts would be broken one day.
Why God choose to challenge your mind - late in your journey here,
I've tried to understand but it only brings more tears.
For the young ones, they don't understand - never will know,
That Mom that always loved us – and never failed to show.
So as today we gather to honor your days with us,
I can only say Thank You, I Love You and in God I do trust.
You've earned your angel wings from the first breath you took,
Your name, Mary, is at the top - the first - in Jesus' book.
I will so miss you, Mom, with all of my heart,
Your gentleness, your dry sense of humor - so many parts.
But I know you will watch over all of us - every single day,
Because that was how you loved us – there's no other way.
So, all ….in closing this poem,
I know Mom has gone to her much-earned new home.
It's all of us still here that need to be strong in our love,

*For Mom…and Pop….and Sandy…and Jaimee, will be watching….
from above.

I Love you, Mom
C. Emery

Comments from Others

Craig Stafford: "Beautiful Mom. Looks like she's ready for Mardi Gras."

*Cheryl Emery - Momma wore these beads every day since last Memorial Day (started with red, white and blue and has steadily increased since then) :). She received them at the Chesapeake Beach Red, White and Blue Festival. Who knew, when she received those free tokens of patriotism, that we would bury them with her. She would never take them off. New ones just got added to them.

Laura Adams Langston -"I find them gloriously funny- I'm warped like that. And a sense of humor will save your sanity.... "

Barbara Hall Gioffre – "Loved to read about your "Momma Chuckles." My Mom also suffered from Alzheimer's. Took care of her for 15 Years."

Pia Evans –" I'm so glad I got to meet your momma. She had to be an amazing mom to raise such a wonderful, loving daughter. Hugs to you."

Juanita Swindell - "We Love "our" Momma's Chuckles!"

Cathy O'Donnell Maida - "Your Momma is a hoot!"

Gloria Bunting - "I also can see the humor in Momma's comments. My Mom passed in July from complications of dementia. God bless you for all you have done. I know it's not easy. PLEASE keep sharing Momma's chuckles. Therapy comes in many forms. Laughter being the best of all. xoxox"

Sharon Hall Reeves - "I enjoy every post about your Mom. It is heartwarming to know that you have managed to keep your sense of humor throughout everything that had been thrown at you!

Heather Wascher – " Momma, many days you were the only chuckle I had. I came to look forward to what you were going to say next. It's funny cuz I never met you, yet felt like I knew you so well...I'll miss my momma chuckles."

Samantha Simms – "Gosh I'm going to miss her sense of humor! She truly could make any "bad" day better."

Jim Davis – "Cheryl, you have my sympathies. I know your heart is hurting right now. As the days pass, surround yourself with family and friends who love you so that their love may push the sadness off to the side. Thank you for sharing your mom with all of us thru "Momma Chuckles" and reminding us that we can find a silver lining if we look for it. ((Hugs))"

I want to give an **Extra Special Thank You** to Daphne Wilson for her reminder. When I recently said, sadly, "I need a Momma Chuckle." She said, ..."Close your eyes .... open your heart.... and listen.... Now, open up your eyes......"

"Momma's chuckles are everywhere."

I Understand

How difficult it must be for you.
To watch me to become less of the person you once knew.
My body is here, but my mind is not.
Things we once shared, I may have forgot.
This will be our longest goodbye.
For the mind of the person you love, is slowing and will die.
I will not act or behave like the person I once was.
But please remember, it's not something I have control of.
I'm sorry for this burden I put on you.
There will be some rough days, with teary eyes and hearts of blue.
But let the love of so many years carry us the rest of the way.
Because this is not forever, and our souls will meet again one day.

~ Joy Rembert (By Permission)

"There will come a time when your loved one will be gone, and you will find comfort in the fact that you were their caregiver."
~ Karen Coetzer (By Permission)

ALZ.org

About the Author

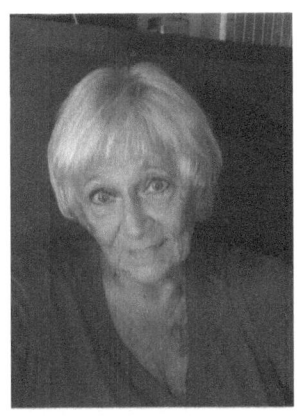

Cheryl was one of numerous caregivers honored to care for her Momma, Mary Haudenshild Jacobs Kirkwood. She lives in Owings, Md. She loves writing, photography, risk-taking adventures and her family. The prior 5 years have been difficult. Losing her Pop 4/14/12; her sister, Sandy 8/31/14; her young niece, Jaimee 3/5/16 and her beautiful Momma, Mary 7/9/16. She wrote this book to help with the needed healing of a Family. She hopes that other caregivers will benefit from "Momma Chuckles", as they love and care for those that need them. It's a rough journey, but she wouldn't have had it any other way. She would travel it again, tomorrow, with her Momma.

This is Cheryl's first book at the age of 66.

Visit her at https://www.facebook.com/cheryl.emery1
Or
https://www.facebook.com/groups/721870717901253/
(Momma Chuckles)
Or
CherylEmery@comcast.net

www.ingramcontent.com/pod-product-compliance
Lightning Source LLC
Chambersburg PA
CBHW030527290526
45786CB00004B/1648